Entwined

ARTHRITIS: MANAGE IT OR ELIMINATE IT

Grandma Mary's Book

Also By Holly Fourchalk

Adrenal Fatigue: Why am I so tired all the time?

Are you what you eat? Why Your Intestines Are The Foundation of Good Health

Cancer: Why what you don't know about your treatment could harm you.

Depression: The Real Cause May Be Your Body.

Diabetes: What Your Physician Doesn't Know

Glutathione: Your Body's Secret Healing Agent

Your Heart: Are you taking care of it?

Inflammation: The Silent Killer

Managing Your Weight: Why your body may be working against you and what you can do about it

The Chocolate Controversy: The Bad, the Mediocre and the Awesome

So What's the Point: If You Have Ever Asked

Your Immune System: Is Yours Protecting You?

Your Vital Liver: How to protect your liver from life's toxins

The Entwined Collection

Entwined: A Romantic Journey Back into Health

Entwined: The Ongoing Journey

Entwined: A Love that Crosses Time

Tom's Collection

The Cosmic Socialite

Cosmic Healing

Cosmic Lessons

All of the above are available at DrHollyBooks.com

Entwined

ARTHRITIS: MANAGE IT OR ELIMINATE IT

Grandma Mary's Book

Holly Fourchalk

PhD., DNM®, RHT, AAP

Cover design by Peter Forde. Published by Vector
Catalyst.

Choices Unlimited for Health & Wellness
Dr. Holly Fourchalk, Ph.D., DNM®, RHT, HT
Tel: 604.764.5203
Websites: www.ChoicesUnlimited.ca
       www.DrHollyBooks.com
E-mail: holly@choicesunlimited.ca

ISBN 978-1-989420-04-1 (softcover)
ISBN 978-1-989420-05-8 (eBook)

Disclaimer

Every effort has been made by the author to ensure that the information in this book is as accurate as possible. However, it is by no means a complete or exhaustive examination of all information.

The author knows what worked for her and what has worked for others, but no two people are the same and so the author cannot and does not render judgment or advice regarding a particular individual.

Further, because our bodies are unique any two individuals may experience different results from the same therapy.

The author believes in both prevention and the superiority of a natural non-invasive approach over drugs and surgery.

The information collected within comes from a variety of researchers and sources from around the world. This information has been accumulated in the Western healing arts over the past thirty years.

Research has shown that one of the top three leading causes of death in North America occurs because of the physician/pharmaceutical component of the scenario.

Perhaps the real leading cause of death and disability is a result of the lack of awareness of natural therapies. These therapies are well known to prevent and treat many common degenerative, inflammatory and oxidative diseases.

The author loves to research and loves to teach. This book is another attempt to increase awareness about health and the many options we have to bring the body back into a healthy balance.

Ever-increasing numbers of people are aware of healing foods and herbs, supplements and modalities but there are still far too many who are not. The fact that our physicians are part of this latter group makes healing even more challenging, yet we are now seeing more and more laboratories around the world and more universities in and outside of the U.S. studying herbs, nutrition and various healing modalities with phenomenal success.

The unfortunate fact is, those who can profit from sickness and disease promote ignorance and the results are devastating.

It is not the intent of the author that anyone should choose to read this book and make decisions regarding their health or medical care based on ideas contained in this book.

It is the responsibility of the individual to find a health care practitioner to work with to achieve optimal health.

The author and publisher are not responsible for any adverse effects or consequences resulting from the use of any of the suggestions or information contained in the book but offer this material as information that the public has a right to hear and utilize at its own discretion.

To my Parents

For all their support and encouragement
My Dad for his ever-listening ear
My Mother for her open mind

Contents

Preface

Before we explore what, The Entwined Collection is about, let's begin by understanding where Dr. Holly is coming from; and how and why she wants everyone to benefit.

Dr. Holly was born with a genetic disorder. Her delivery was a confusion of issues that went wrong; some of which were not recognized at the time. Her petite mal, or absence, seizures started when she was 4 years old, though nobody recognized what was happening. Absence seizures are named for the brief loss of consciousness, and often misinterpreted as daydreaming.

At the age of nine, she was in a dramatic accident which provoked, and accelerated, her female development. It also provoked the myoclonic seizures which manifested themselves in powerful twitches or muscle jerks or spasms. By the time she was 14, the petite mal seizures and myoclonic seizures now included grand mal, or tonic-clonic, seizures.

The grand mal/tonic-clonic seizures, a type of generalized seizure, affected the entire brain. During these types of seizures, she would lose consciousness and the skeletal muscles would thrash violently and uncontrollably followed by amnesia, headaches, a damaged tongue and exhaustion.

After Holly's first grand mal seizure, her mother found her passed out on the floor and was devastated. She had already lost two children; she was not prepared to lose another. The problem became more complex. The more medication Holly was put on, the more seizures she had; never mind all the weight and other issues the medications caused. Four, five, six mornings out of seven she woke up with petite mal and myoclonic seizures. The medical profession blamed the car accident and increased both the number of drugs and their dosage, which of course provoked more seizures.

Struggling to resolve the seizures, her mother attended medical conferences, even though she didn't understand half of what they were saying. She booked Holly into Naturopaths, Reflexologists, and Acupuncturists, and anyone who thought they could stop the seizures. They even worked with Edgar Cayce remedies. They had to find a way to stop the seizures.

It wasn't until Holly was studying neurological issues in university that she recognized she had been having seizures since she was four years old.

Holly's favorite and most beloved practitioner was Dr. Loffler, an Osteopath/Naturopath, whom she started to see at the age of 18. He identified a number of issues compounding the problem going back to the car accident. Her second favorite physician was the neurologist she started see at the age of 26. She identified the genetic issue that was causing the seizures and other problems. Holly learned that people with this type of disorder didn't usually graduate from high school and were usually dead by the time they were 26 years old. In addition, her EEGs indicated she shouldn't be able to talk.

In university she was diagnosed with an ovarian tumor the size of a hard ball. She was told she needed surgery immediately as it was dangerous. Dr. Loffler, however, put her on a specific diet for ovarian tumors. Due to family pressure, she underwent a second laparotomy 3.5 weeks later. The tumor was gone. Her medical doctors never asked how she accomplished that.

At the age of 26, she burnt her eyes and the specialist told her she had to join classes to learn how to be blind as she would be legally blind by the time she was 30. She went back a year and half later with 20/19 vision. He never asked how she accomplished that.

In school, Dr. Holly had to deal with issues like ADD (Attention Deficit Disorder) and Dyslexia, yet she studied hard and diligently and always maintained her honor roll marks. She loved numbers and went into university hoping to get degrees in Physics and Math and become an Astrophysicist. However, that wasn't the plan life had for her and she came out as a Registered Psychologist. She ran her own practice for some 20 years.

During her training and practice as a psychologist, she was constantly frustrated at the total lack of training regarding the nutrients the brain required to function properly. Many of her clients came in with issues of depression and anxiety and other disorders. Dr. Holly would often suggest they see other practitioners like Naturopaths, Herbalists, or go for Hydro colonics. Repeatedly, supposed psychological issues were successfully solved, using other healing disciplines.

Dr. Holly attended Medical School as part of her of her first PhD, *PsychoNeuroEndocrinology*, which was in research and design. Two of the professors asked her to please stop asking questions. Why? Utilizing her knowledge in research and design; she repeatedly pointed out that referenced studies were not proving what they claimed. In fact, most of "evidenced based medicine" was not in fact, evidenced based – it was hypothesis based AND more and more of the hypotheses were being proven wrong. This was destroying the moral of the students.

Subsequently she learned how Big Pharma controls most Medical School Curriculums; and the Protocol and Procedure MDs are required to follow. In addition, they are now saying it can take up to 40 years for good research to get to the MDs and to the hospitals.

One thing Dr. Holly was never short on, was energy. Consequently, in addition to her academic profession and Psychology practice, Dr. Holly also opened and ran a big rig trucking company; an accounting business; a warehouse and distribution business and a rental company. However, she found herself challenged with the lack of morals and integrity in the trucking and warehousing businesses and eventually went back to school.

Dr. Holly got fed up with the limitations imposed on her within the field of psychology and enrolled in Naturopathic College. It was a double graduate program, 8 years completed in 4 years. Dr. Holly was also required to complete two years of Premed during the first year; meanwhile she continued her Psychology Practice.

By the time second year started, the seizures started up again. Very Scary. She hadn't had seizures for 15 years. In addition, other major health issues evolved. Her body kept telling her to quit. Holly was never a quitter. However, the College found out she was having seizures and put her on hold for a year. When she returned the following year, the seizures started up within three weeks, so she transferred from the Naturopathic program to a Doctor of Natural Medicine, wherein she could go at her own pace.

Holly went to India to complete, and intern for, for two Ayurveda medical programs. She also completed a Masters in Herbal Medicine: *Bridging Ayurveda, Traditional Chinese Medicine and Western Herbal Medicine*. She studied homeopathy and reflexology, locally and abroad. She then applied and was accepted for a PhD program in Nutrition where she received a Cum Laude for her thesis identifying the biochemistry of cellular healing.

During this time, Dr. Holly applied to, and was accepted, into Law School. She wanted to know the ins and outs of law to protect practitioners from their Colleges and from Big Pharma.

While completing the various degrees, Dr. Holly worked with a mentor as she prepared to leave the College of Psychologists. In the meantime, the College of Psychologists accused her of practicing "non-evidence based' medicine. She volunteered to provide workshops teaching the nutrients that the brain required to function from a nutritional and biochemistry perspective, but they were not interested. She left.

Her practice as a Dr. of Natural Medicine was up and running by this time. She published twelve books for the general public over the next four years. She wanted the general public to understand the differences between Conventional Medicine/managing symptoms and REAL medicine/resolving the underlying issues.

The Entwined Collection
One day Dr. Holly woke up with an idea. Write a sexy romantic novel that would attract a larger audience, incorporating a huge amount of health information explaining REAL medicine and *Entwined: A Romantic Journey Back into Health* came to fruition.

Preparing to go away on a vacation and write the sequel to *Entwined*, Dr. Holly woke up with the idea of the Round Table and asking each character in the book to write their own book. This way, she could a use all the different literary genres to convey a huge amount of information on health and wellness. People could enjoy learning about REAL health and medicine reading the writing genre they preferred: educational, romantic, mystery, political, etc. Consequently, each book in the Entwined Book Collection is written with a different slant and from a different perspective according to the character of the Entwined Book Project responsible for the book.

Dr. Holly attributes different healing disciplines to each of the Gibson family members who all work at the Gibson Clinic. With two exceptions: Dr. Holly is not a physiotherapist, and nor did she finish her Traditional Chinese Medicine program. Otherwise, Dr. Holly has all the degrees and designations to professionally address the issues focused on by her characters.

On a personal note, **"Entwined"** has a lot more meaning for Dr. Holly than just being the collection of books resulting from *Entwined: A Romantic Journey Back into Health*. The word Entwined reflects life itself. All aspects of our beingness are entwined: from the moral/ethical; to the spiritual/religious; to the intellectual/emotional; to the physical/sexual; to the family/social; to the ingestion/elimination; and to all the different energetics. They are all **entwined**. In addition, the individual is entwined with their family; with their social network; with the community; and with the nation. Again, all is **entwined;** encompassing the local to the universal. Nothing happens in isolation;

entwined embraces all, whether local or all matter stretching throughout the universe.

Consequently, when we look at our health and wellbeing, we need to take the whole being into consideration. To isolate any aspect of our being, whether it be our physical health, psychological health, energetic health, etc. is to negate an aspect of who we are.

Two powerful words for Dr. Holly are **Entwined** and **Choices**. Just as our health is immeasurably **entwined** with all of whom we are; so are all our **Choices Entwined** with what we choose to do with those choices. Whether it is our symptoms, our health, our relationships, our careers, etc., we can choose to manage, or we can choose to eliminate. The **CHOICE** is ours.

All of us involved in the writing, editing, publishing and marketing of these books, hope you enjoy the books; learn a lot from the books; and wish you the very best of health.

In Grandma Mary's book, *Arthritis: Manage or Eliminate It*, listen to Grandma Mary and how her life changed after she was diagnosed with arthritis. Discover how the pain killers and arthritis destroyed her life and, more importantly, how she resolved the arthritis and got her life back. When she met the Gibsons, she learned about the different types of arthritis; the causes of arthritis; and finally, how to eliminate her arthritis.

Each book in the Entwined Collection is required to focus on health and wellness. So, Grandma Mary, tells her story of healing simply and beautifully from her Grandma's perspective.

Chapter 1

Where it all began

I could say it all began when my arthritis started, but that's not really true.

Obviously, that's when my arthritis began. BUT this book began with my daughter. You see, I have one of those daughters that never stops questioning.

Little kids ask a pile of questions. You give them an easy answer, and they are off and running again.

But not my Maria. The child wanted to know the why to the why to the why and she couldn't be distracted with simple answers. She really wanted to know. When she was a young one, I spent half of my time in the libraries trying to find answers for her incessant questions.

When she was 12 years old, the pastor of the church phoned me to ask "Where does she get these questions? No one else in the congregation even thinks to ask these kinds of questions."

But the questions didn't stop in childhood, or in adolescence, or in young adulthood. In fact, she is nearly 50 and still comes up with a ton of questions that most people never even consider. Some people never grow out of having temper tantrums, my Maria never grew out of asking questions.

So why would I say that Maria's incessant questions became the origins of this book?

Well Maria started this Breakfast Philosophy thing on Sunday mornings. It's a Pot Luck Breakfast open to everyone who enjoys discussions – philosophical, psychological, spiritual, whatever. Most Sunday mornings, people come. She may have a group of 5 to 6 or she may have a group of 25 to 30. One never knows who will join. But it is always interesting.

I love the discussions and I enjoy the socializing that comes with them.

Then, this one Sunday, Maria wakes up with this brilliant idea of asking everyone who showed up: "If you had to write a book what kind of book would you write and what about?

Some people decided that would write a history or political book, others said they would write a romance, some liked other types of novels, like sci-fi or mystery, an autobiography or an educational book. Of course, some said 'no way', they didn't want to write any kind of book.

In the end, we all agreed to write a book, the only common theme was that they all had to be about health. It didn't matter how it involved health – as long as it did.

Well of course, my answer was an educational book on how to eliminate arthritis.

Why? Again, you may ask. Good question, and that is the point of this book.

I am 75 years old this year and I have suffered with both Osteo and Rheumatoid Arthritis for over 25 years. I have taken all types of pain killers prescribed to me. Some worked for a period of time, some didn't work at all. Many are addictive and dangerous. Many harm other parts of your body causing even more problems! Most drugs, of every kind, deplete the body of nutrients!! Half of the most commonly prescribed drugs can cause cancer!!!

I lived with arthritis for many years. I know how it limits your life. Actually, how it changes your life. Whether it starts slowly or develops overnight, arthritis has a huge impact on our lives in a wide variety of ways.

Pain robs you of everything!

On a physical level, the stiffness and the pain have a huge impact on what we do. Our days become more and more restricted as activities become more and more painful.

I stopped all the baking that I had done for years. The arthritis in my hands made baking a painful activity.

I stopped going to my grandchildren's various programs, art presentations, dance competitions, etc. because sitting for any length of time was simply too painful.

I used to quickly shower and get on with my day. The arthritis required that I sit in an Epsom salt bath, hoping the pain would disappear.

I used to go for long walks everyday with my husband. The walks got shorter and shorter until eventually, I just didn't go. It was simply too painful.

Arthritis can also have a huge impact on your romantic life. My husband and I used to laugh about how fortunate we were that we both enjoyed our physical relationship even as senior citizens. As the arthritis progressed, it was just too painful to engage physically.

The family physician said I should keep up a minimum amount of exercise, it was important to the body. Sorry, not with the pain I was suffering. At first, I struggled to overcome it and push my way through it, but eventually, I just stopped. I understood that my body needed movement and activity to stay healthy. But what was the cost?

When we restrict our day to day activities because it is too painful to do them, this then impacts on a body in a number of ways. Our bodies need to be actively physically engaged in life for a wide variety of health reasons. When we don't provide this movement to the body, there is a domino effect that can lead to various other health issues.

The pain from the arthritis, and I would assume, any kind of pain, is exhausting. One of the issues that can be affected is our sleep. When you can't get comfortable at night, you have a difficult time sleeping.

Sleeping, I learned, is where the body does most of its healing. That deep sleep is essential for good health. But I couldn't sleep. So, I went back to the physician who put me on sleeping pills.

Well, it turns out the sleeping pills prevent the deeper stages of sleep where all the healing occurs. But it does give you the sense that you were asleep.

When you are prevented from getting a good healthy sleep, your body is not able to do the repair work it needs to do. But if we don't take the sleeping pills, we simply get more and more tired. Along with the increasing pain, we end up with fatigue in each system: emotional, physical, and psychological.

Pain even affects us mentally. Pain can make it difficult to think and concentrate. It can actually affect our memory capacity.

I found this embarrassing. I used to have a good memory. Now increasingly I couldn't remember names, where I put things, or what I supposed to do that day. I laughed that eventually I wasn't going to be able to remember my name. The humor was a cover up for my rapidly developing fear.

I didn't want to tell the family physician about my loss of memory because I was afraid he would now diagnose me with Alzheimer's. I knew that not only came along with more prescription drugs, but also in my mind, it was the end of me. Another fear.

We will often make decisions too fast because of the pain. When in fact, we should take the time to explore different options. But the pain gets in our way. We make decisions that help us to accommodate the pain rather than effective decisions for our lives.

Our emotions can also be affected by pain. We can become:

- Anxious
- Depressive
- Easily frustrated
- Impatient
- Irritable
- Intolerant
- Moody
- Reactive

Our emotions may 'ride' on the surface. The pain, lack of sleep, and well-being can cause depression-like symptoms. We may also go into a state of despair – with there never being an end in sight, with losing a sense of hope, and feeling a lack of control over anything in our lives.

Again, I was afraid to tell my family physician about it, because I didn't want to get another diagnosis of depression and have to go on anti-depressants.

I was fortunate, my family didn't push me to go to the family physician and they didn't want me to take more pills. Instead, my daughter and her husband built a lovely suite in the basement of their home and we moved in there.

Unfortunately, too many seniors are pushed to go to the physician, collect even more prescription drugs, which cause more symptoms and waste more money. They even now have a term for this accumulation of prescriptions, cocktail drugs.

When you can't move and you can't think and you can't remember, you end up spending more and more time alone. The more time alone you spend, the more isolated you become, and the easier it is to go into a deeper depressive state.

For me, my emotions were always near the surface. I was exhausted from not getting enough sleep and frustrated that I couldn't resolve the pain. When I finally mentioned my depression to my MD, he wanted me to go on anti-depressants. I simply said, "No, I didn't think it was necessary." The practitioners at the Gibson's Clinic told me – frustration and depression are two entirely different things. They advised, "Don't get conned into taking anti-depressants. I found this great book called *Depression: The Real Cause may be in Your Body*.

But those aren't the only issues. On a nutritional level, we not only loose our appetite but it may often become physically more and more difficult to prepare foods. As much as I stopped baking, I still did most of our cooking. I was lucky again, because my daughter, Maria, also brought down a lot of cooking and baking for us. But many seniors, especially those who live on their own, don't get the good, healthy meals. Or they order meals to be delivered from conglomerates. While I am sure those companies do try hard, it just isn't the same as home-made cooking.

So, between getting less nutrients in the body and the medications depleting nutrients in the body, the body is able to accommodate less and less, and other problems start to emerge.

Again, for me this was a little different. As I said. my husband and I live in the basement suite of my daughter Maria and her husband Duncan. Maria is a real health nut who is always making sure that my husband and I not only got good nutrients, but she would also make my favorite scones for me. It is great when you have a supportive family, but you really do need to go beyond that and solve the actual problem.

Then of course, there is the damage caused by the pain killers. Did you know that pain killers can actually *increase chronic pain*?

Some can destroy the lining of your stomach – which can cause pain in and of itself. NSAIDS (Non-steroidal anti-inflammatory drugs) can cause small erosions in the stomach even after a single dosage! And, they can cause other gut issues. And, they can increase your blood pressure! And, they can cause problems with your kidneys.

Acetaminophen is easier on the stomach than NSAIDs but can damage the liver!!

COX-2 inhibitors are supposed to be a better category of NSAIDs (Nonsteroidal Anti-inflammatory Drugs) but they can be hard on the heart!! And, of course, increase your blood pressure. But let's not forget, they can also do a number on your kidneys! Oh dear.

Many types of pain killers are addictive, some cause increased risk of heart attack, and others cause liver damage. Some can make you suicidal! Oh dear, why not just eliminate the arthritis?

On a different level, some people end up spending the whole of their day just accommodating the pain. Learning to move around it. Learning different pain management or pain control methods. Some people go to pain clinics struggling to learn how to work around the pain. Ultimately, pain becomes the center of their lives at cost to everything and everyone else.

WOW!! Yes, if you hadn't thought of it before – pain does rob our lives from us. I didn't realize how much my whole life had suffered because of the pain, simply because I was so focused on the pain. Until the big event.

A miracle happened. This daughter of mine told me I needed to see this family of practitioners at the Gibson's Clinic. I am going to tell you about this family further into the book. But in the meantime, she was sure they could help me. For me, I was in so much constant pain, I was willing to see anyone.

And today? Well I have no swelling, no pain, and I have full use of my hands again! The arthritis was also in my knees and feet. It had started to move into my back, but it was predominantly in my hands. Now, thanks to the Gibson's Clinic, the pain is entirely gone. Not just the pain but also the inflammation, the redness, the irregular joints – it is all gone!!!

I am off all the medications and went on a special diet that allowed my cognitive and emotional functioning return to normal.

In other words, I have my life back. That is so huge. I am so grateful. Consequently, I decided to write a book for you and give you the CHOICE as well. The CHOICE between managing your arthritis and eliminating it!

So, in a sense this first chapter of the book gives you both the origins of the book and the final chapter, all in one. So, what is the rest of the book about?

What I am going to do for you in this book is provide:

1) An understanding of arthritis;
2) An understanding of the causes of arthritis;
3) An understanding of why prescription drugs don't ultimately work; and
4) An understanding of why REAL medicine DOES ultimately work.

It is my desire that by the end of this book, you will understand why I no longer have arthritis and that YOU too can follow the path that the Gibsons walked me down. You do have CHOICES in your life and you too choose to: **Manage** Your Arthritis OR **Eliminate** Your Arthritis.

I hope, for your sake, you decide to take the road I took because life is hugely different when you are not always working around the pain and limitations caused from arthritis.

Chapter 2

An Understanding of Arthritis

Now this part may not be for you. But it was important to the Gibsons and it turned out to be important to me.

I found that the more you understand about the affliction you suffer from, the more you can help your body eliminate it. Perhaps that is why some people think that the mind is so powerful.

Just think about the 'placebo effect'. It is so powerful, it can account for 32-38% of the results in a given study. That is powerful. Now, if we can add onto the 'placebo effect' by understanding what is going on in our bodies and helping the process…wouldn't that be even better?

Well, I think so. So, you have your first CHOICE: you can read this next part and learn about the different kinds of arthritis and how they evolve, or you can skip it.

If a 75-year-old woman with only a high school education can learn this stuff and even write about it, then believe me, you will have no problem.

So, let's figure this stuff out.

First, did you know that there are over 100 different conditions involving your joints? That's a lot, don't you think?

There are, however, only three major categories of arthritis:

1) Rheumatoid and Psoriatic arthritis – these are thought to be auto-immune disorders – and yes, we can eliminate them.
2) Septic arthritis – which evolves from an infection in the joint and may actually be gout.
3) Osteo arthritis – which involves joint degeneration for almost any reason – that can include the bones, cartilage, ligaments, etc.

There are also some other not so common categories like:

4) Spondylarthritis – usually affects joints of the spine. This type of inflammation in the connective tissues in the spine is called entheses.
5) Ankylosing spondylitis – also refers to joints of the spine. This is where excess calcium causes calcium deposits or new bone growths. Pain

usually occurs later in the night and into the morning.

6) Psoriatic arthritis - another autoimmune condition. This usually occurs in people who already suffer from psoriasis but not necessarily.

7) Reiter's syndrome or reactive arthritis – usually occurs in the feet and lower extremities and usually follows a GIT or urinary tract infection.

In addition, bacteria can cause arthritis. A common one is Staphylococcus aureus or staph. But there are also viral and fungal infections that can cause arthritis and we need to build the immune system to deal with that as opposed to simply take pain killers. These ones usually involve the knee or the hips, ankles or writs.

I even found out that disseminated gonococcal infection or DGI caused by a bacterium. The Neisseria gonorrhoeae bacteria can lead to arthritic conditions.

A more common bacterial infection we get from hospitals, this acquired bacteremia can predate the onset of the arthritis by day, weeks or months – and you didn't even know it. But the still put you on pain killers rather than find out the cause and eliminate the cause – that they caused!!!

I certainly don't remember my family physician checking for all of these possibilities.

In addition, there are a number of diagnoses that mimic arthritic conditions, but need to be correctly diagnosed: lupus, fibromyalgia, polymyalgia, back pain and tendinopathy.

I found a couple of pictures on the internet, of what a healthy joint versus an unhealthy joint look like to give you an idea of what might be going in your body.

So, this first picture is a nice healthy joint.

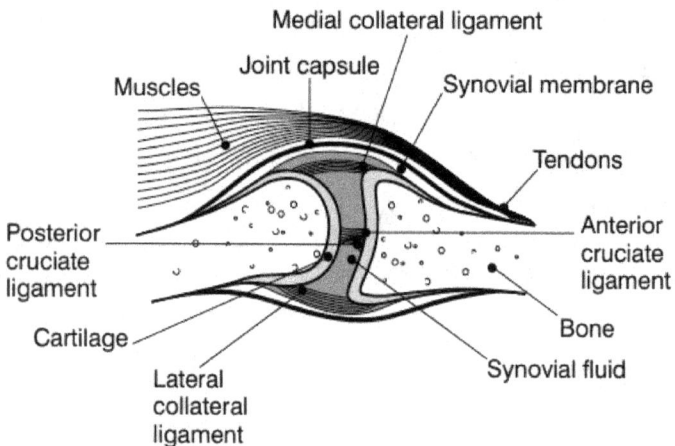

These next pictures are some different ways of seeing very unhealthy joints.

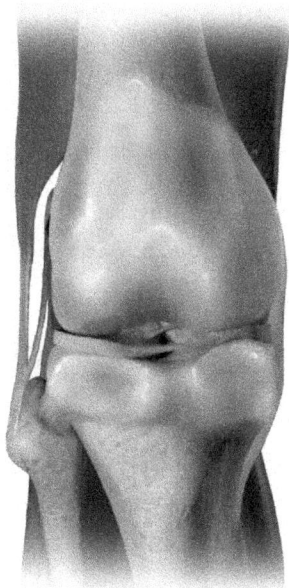

Healthy Joint   *Unhealthy Joint*

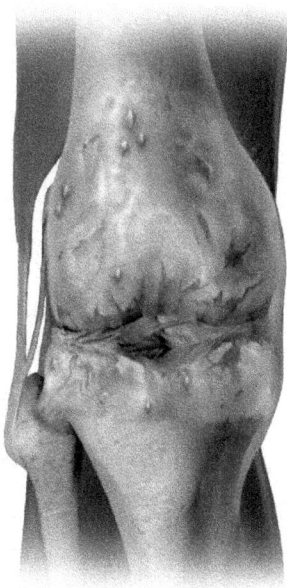

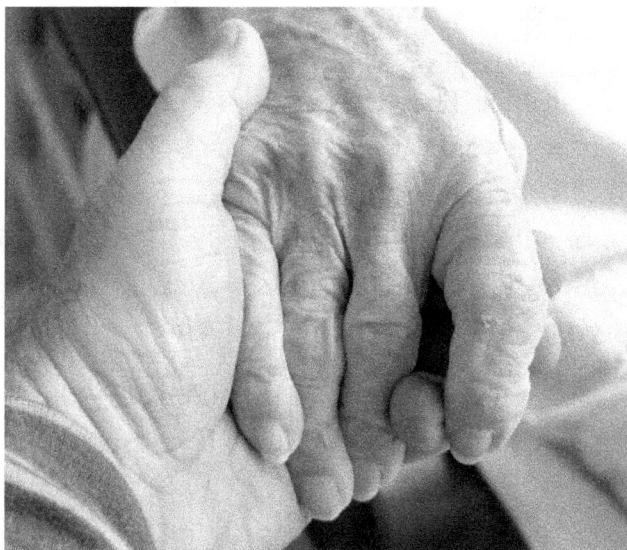

But how do these different conditions arise? That's what I wanted to know. Yeah, I know. My daughter comes by it naturally. I too, ask a lot of questions. But it was fun to blame it on my daughter.

How come I had arthritis and my husband, or my best friend didn't? What I had done wrong along life's pathway that caused me to have arthritis. I was certainly glad that they didn't have to suffer like I did but WHY was I suffering.

The MDs just said it was part of 'Old Age'. Well, if it was part of 'Old Age' why didn't everyone have it? I thought we were supposed to enjoying the 'Golden Years'? From my perspective, it was the 'Painful Years' not the 'Golden Years'.

When I asked my MDs how I could eliminate the arthritis, they said I couldn't. And for years, unfortunately, I actually believed them. They were the physicians. They were supposed to be smart and know everything. So, before we go any further, I want to share something with you. You know those big medical journals they talk about? Where they publish the medical studies. Well, let me tell you something about them.

First off, for years now they are full of Big Pharma advertising and very little in the way of research.

Secondly, the articles have to be accepted by the Editors – who represent Big Pharma – so that tells you write off the top what is going to get accepted and what isn't.

Thirdly, you pay to have your research published, so if the research showed negative or neutral results – which is most of the research – they don't get published.

Fourthly, the Editor-in-Chief of two of the most prestigious medical journals, the Lancet and the New England Journal of Medicine, recently made the following statements.

First, we have the Lancet:

> "The case against science is straightforward; much of the scientific literature, perhaps half, may simply be untrue. Afflicted by studies with small sample sizes, tiny effects, invalid exploratory analysis, and flagrant conflicts of interest, together with an obsession for pursuing fashionable trends of dubious importance, science has taken a turn towards darkness."[1]

And then from the New England Journal of Medicine, Dr Marcia Angell wrote:

> "It is simply no longer possible to believe much of the clinical research that is published, or to rely on the judgement of trusted physicians or authoritative medical guidelines. I take no

pleasure in this conclusion, which I reached slowly and reluctantly over my two decades as an editor of the New England Journal of Medicine."[2]

Wow! That is huge. Even the Chief Editors are admitting that both the research and the trusted authorities are not to be trusted. Where does that leave us? Well, it leaves us turning to REAL medicine. Real food and herbs and getting to the source of the problem, rather than managing symptoms with synthetic drugs.

Oh dear, I am getting beyond myself here. So, let's back up a bit.

I am going to identify the three most commonly held beliefs about the causes of arthritis in Western culture…and then I am going to go out on a limb and explain some of the Eastern beliefs, for interest sake. Myself? I was happy enough to work with the Western beliefs. But if we are going to write a book about it, I thought I should include as much as I have learned. So, let's get started.

The first group I am going to look at is the most superficial group:

Inflammatory Conditions

I say this is the most superficial because it is the most obvious aspect of arthritis. The area of the body that is suffering is inflamed. It is inflamed and inflammation hurts.

I read a lot of stuff on the internet these days about how inflammation is the root cause of most disorders and dysfunctions in today's society. Or how most of the conditions that people go to an MD for today, are inflammation based. You have probably heard or read similar kinds of statements.

Well, in my mind that isn't telling us anything. We need to know what is causing the inflammation before we can really solve it. And this is where I believe a lot of Conventional medicine goes sideways. Yes, they can give you pain killers and anti-inflammatories, or you can take a variety of different 'over the counter' or OTCs drugs. BUT they do not solve the problem. They are only trying to manage the symptoms.

This is one reason that I am now such a big fan of REAL medicine. All the different healing practices or disciplines or modalities, whatever you want to call them, that look at what is causing the problem and work at resolving the cause of the problem rather than managing the symptoms.

Just think, when prescription drugs are simply managing the problem, you end up on the drugs indefinitely which is great for Big Pharma. You get to the source of the problem and eliminate it –

your life comes back to you and you keep your money. Not so good for Big Pharma.

Anyways, let me re-emphasize here, just saying that the cause of the majority of problems are inflammatory based is as informative as saying that "the only true cause of death is birth". It really doesn't tell us anything. So, let's look further and get a brief overview of the different causes of inflammation. Note, I said 'brief' AND I am going to deal with issues only in terms of arthritis.

Causes of Inflammation

1) Infection – this is thought to be the basis of Rheumatoid arthritis – but it actually goes way beyond that and we will expand on it.
2) Toxicity – there are so many different types that we are going to have a whole section on this.
3) Trauma to the body, for example, any kind of physical injury like a broken bone.
4) Prescription drugs – yes, the drugs that your MD prescribes for you and/or those OTCs can cause arthritic conditions – can you believe it? I bet this section will be a real eye opener for you.
5) Dehydration – now I thought dehydration simply meant that I wasn't drinking enough water. I am sure you have heard the 8x8 rule: we need to drink 8, 8 oz., glasses of water a day

– well it turns out that can be dangerous. There are issues, however, that come into why we are so dehydrated, and I look forward to explaining them to you.

6) Auto-immune disease – that is when our body thinks our own cells or tissues are the problem and starts to eliminate them – again, this can actually be reversed. Do you know that auto-immune diseases can be caused by pathogens in your teeth and gums? We will discuss this further in Chapter 8.

That all sounds pretty straight forward, doesn't it? But there is a lot more to it than that and we are going to go through it all, one step at a time so you get a good understanding.

Chapter 3

Causes of Inflammation: Infection

Okay, so hopefully you stayed with me while I explained arthritis. Now, the next five chapters are going to deal with the causes of inflammation. We all know that inflammation is a huge component of arthritis – so let's figure what causes it. You will be very surprised at some of the information here.

Did you know that we are constantly being infected? Let's look at some of the ways that we get infected:

- By the atmosphere that surrounds our skin;
- By the air we breathe;
- By the water we drink; and
- By the food we eat.

Wow, virtually anything and everything that keeps us alive is also full of infection causing critters. They critters are called pathogens. They come in a wide variety of forms, like:

- Viruses;

- Bacteria;
- Mold and yeast; and
- Worms.

But Antibiotics are Supposed to Protect Us

In the old days, we thought that antibiotics would take care of these things and we would live forever. But as I am sure you know, we are moving past the era of antibiotics.

Did you know that over 80% of the antibiotics in North America are found in our food? So, whether you are taking them with a prescription or not, the likelihood is that you are ingesting them.

We have heard a lot in the last decade, about how there is over-use and abuse with MDs prescribing way too many antibiotics. For instance, they are prescribed for viruses – when they are only meant for bacteria. Further, they should only be utilized in severe cases, not for everything. Why?

There are a huge number of reasons, but let's go over just two important ones.

1) Bacteria and DNA

Bacteria can change their DNA. And they can do it quickly. For instance, some can even change their DNA within 15 minutes! That contributes to why some bacteria are so adept at accommodating to the antibiotics and why we are finding that there is an increasing number of bacteria that antibiotic resistant.

Isn't our immune system meant to deal with these bacteria and other pathogens? Of course, it is. The immune system is kind of like our muscles. It needs all kinds of nutrients in order to stay healthy AND it needs to get a work out in order to keep functioning well.

Think about it. If muscles don't get enough nutrition, they will start to weaken. We also know that if we don't use a muscle it will atrophy or die off. Well, our immune system is similar in that if we keep preventing it from functioning by taking vaccinations, immunizations and antibiotics, then it becomes weakened and it doesn't work when we need it to.

Now some people are going to argue that we need vaccinations and immunizations. And there may be a time and place for them. But when I looked at all the charts that showed the safety and efficacy of these injections, I came out with a different understanding. So, I went and listened to some leading experts in various fields. Not the guys that are paid to give the talks, but the researchers actually doing the work. And again, the research shows that the injections help very few in the long run and harm a tremendous number.

Further, pathogens, that's the bad guys, go in cycles. They come in and have a huge impact and then they die out. Usually by the time injections come on board is when the pathogen is on its way out.

If you want more research on these topics, I've included some links at end of the book. You might also want to look up the difference between Relative Risk and Absolute Risk.[3] It appears that our MDs are being manipulated by Big Pharma as much as we are.

Back to the point in hand, just like when a muscle will atrophy when it is not used, our immune system will also, in effect, atrophy. There is no point for the body to keep something going if we never use it. Now I admit that is not an exact analogy, but it is a good one for our purposes here.

2) Microbiota

The second big issue concerns whether we ingest artificial food or take the synthetic artificial prescriptions, they both destroy a big part of the gut immune system called the microbiota. The microbiota are the good bacteria & other microbes in your gut that work alongside of your immune system.

Maybe you have heard that most of your immune system is found in your gut, well that's true.

However, it also runs throughout your body AND likewise there are good bacteria throughout your body that also support the immune system.

The problem with the antibiotics is that they kill the good guys just like they kill the bad guys. Artificial synthetic medications do not have the capacity to differentiate between good stuff and bad stuff like the REAL medications (food and herbs) can.

Remember, those good guys are important to our immune system. So, when the drugs kill off the good guys, they are also disarming our immune system and our ability to fight anything. And as you can see from the short list above, we need to fight a lot of things all the time.

You are going to find that I side track like that a lot through this book, but I think it is important information for all of us to know.

Now, you can control the amount of antibiotics you ingest by prescription, but what about the antibiotics that are in the very food you eat? Unless you are committed to eating truly organic food, which is difficult, you have no control.

Further, we all know that "Organic" is a loosely defined word and is a very poorly regulated industry. So, do we go back growing our own food? Well, if we are healthy and flexible and not suffering from arthritis, then we might. But for the most part, that is a challenge. However, we can certainly take steps towards resolving the issue and we will show how throughout the book.

So, let's look at how all these pathogens attack our body 24/7.

1) By the atmosphere that surrounds our skin

We know the air is full of pollutants, but it is also full of pathogens. The air surrounds our body. You have already heard that our skin is the largest organ in the body in terms of surface area and weight. That skin organ has three predominant functions:

- Protection;
- Regulation; and
- Sensation.

Actually, I was amazed at how many functions the skin carries out for us.

There is now a National Institute of **Arthritis** and Musculoskeletal and **Skin Diseases.** So, let's look at some basic functions of the skin and then how that pertains to arthritis:

- Your skin helps to keep your musculoskeletal body together.
- Your skin helps to regulate the temperature inside of your body – that is why we sweat.

- Your skin is one of the 4 major pathways to eliminate toxins and pathogens from the body – your breath, stool and urine are the other pathways.
- And of course, your skin protects you from pathogens in the air.
    - But the one that is most important to us here is protection from microorganisms! The skin has different kinds of cells in it. For instance, Langerhans cells, phagocytic cells and epidermal dendritic cells. You can look each kind up if you want, but basically all these kinds of cells protect us from skin infections – infections impact on the immune system – and that can provoke arthritis!!
- Your skin protects you from UVA rays: we need the UVB rays to make Vitamin D. Did you know that the byproducts of making Vitamin D in the skin are anti-carcinogens? Good reason not to put on those dangerous sunscreen lotions – they protect you from the UVB rays that you need and usually don't protect you from the UVA rays that are harmful. Unfortunately, when we put all the man-made creams and makeup and lotions and sunscreen on our skin, it not only weakens the natural skin immunity system BUT all that man-made synthetic toxic

stuff ends up going into the blood vessels that move through our skin – Yuck!

Also, most of the sunscreens are full of toxins! What a world we live in.

- o Did you know that the Vitamin D3 that your skin makes is not really a vitamin? It is actually a hormone.
- o When we take the Vitamin D3 supplement we don't make the anti-carcinogens like we do when our skin makes it.
- o Nonetheless, Vitamin D3 has an impact on about 20% of our DNA.
- o It helps to maintain the proper levels of calcium and phosphorus in our blood, which in turn can be of help to our teeth & gums and our bones.
- o It helps to regulate our cholesterol.
- o It is hugely important to our immune system – yeah that's what we were talking about with regard to causes of arthritis. It helps to protect us against cancers, diabetes, MS and a multitude of other problems.

Research shows that people with arthritis usually have low levels of Vitamin D3 and that low levels increase the risk of both rheumatoid arthritis and osteoarthritis.

Dehydration: yes, our skin protects us from dehydration. It isn't just about the amount of fluid we take in. By the way, did you know that bottled water can be very toxic to the body? The pH of most of the bottled waters is horrible for you. Some even have a pH of 2.2 – that is basically an acid! Again, what a world we live in.

In fact, many people get arthritis and low back pain as a result of being dehydrated. Did you know that heartburn, angina, high blood pressure, migraines, and a variety of other things can also be sign of dehydration? It is good to learn the different causes.

Too often physicians want to put us on pills, when there is a simple solution to the problem.

The skin also protects the inner body from physical injuries/trauma.

So, it starts to become apparent when we want to look after our health and our immune system, we need to be careful with what we put on our skin.

Yes, the bottom line is we need to protect our skin wisely so it can protect us from infections and other issues.

2) By the air we breathe

Yes, we are all aware that the air is polluted, especially in the big cities. But I was amazed to find out that trade winds spread huge amounts of toxins, gases and dangerous pathogens around the world.

The Pacific side of North America, for instance, suffers all the manufacturing toxins in the trade winds from China and Japan. If there are coastal mountains, then the mountains create a wall for many of those toxins to stay in the coastal vicinities.

Regardless of where we live, we are exposed to toxins and pathogens in the very air we breathe. I was talking with a horticultural specialist at a nursery near me. We started to laugh, a very sad laugh. We came to the conclusion that if you wanted to get away from toxins, you might have to live high up in the Himalayan Mountains. Not for me! So, what do we do?

Now MDs would probably argue that your lungs are designed to deal with all of those pathogens. My response back to them is: why do Insurance Companies now have special programs for workers that were exposed to asbestos if our lungs are supposed to deal with the pathogens, never mind tobacco and cancer and I am sure you can think of all kinds of other issues.

The fact of the matter is that when pathogens and toxins accumulations are strong enough OR accumulate for long enough OR some combination of the two, they can weaken our respiratory immune system. And in today's world, the air is full of synthetic toxins, gases, etc., that can destroy our respiratory immune system.

In fact, recent research has shown that cities with the highest levels of pollution particulates have a strong correlation between pollution spikes and rheumatoid arthritis flare ups! US studies have shown that people who live with 50 meters of a highway have a higher incidence of rheumatoid arthritis.

Now, why would this be so? Well, the theory is that in places where the immune system, the environment and genetics meet can be more vulnerable to the damaging effects of the pollutants and can cause rheumatoid arthritis.

Our lungs need an immune system to take care of all the pathogens and pollutants that we breathe in without even being aware of it.

So, the bottom line, is we must take care of our Respiratory System so that it can protect us from the air that we breathe.

3) By the water we drink

We all know that we not only need air to breathe, but we also need water to drink. You may have heard about how toxic our water is. But here are some more interesting facts.

1) Bottled water is in most places worse than tap water. Now I recognize that there are places where you can "light" the tap water with a match, it is so toxic thanks to gas drilling and fracking. So obviously, in places like that people really do benefit from bottled water.
2) Did you know that many of the bottled waters have pH levels of 2.2? So, for those of you who don't know about pH, let me give you a very brief understanding. pH relates to hydrogen and acidity and alkalinity. It goes on a scale of 1- 14 where 7 is neutral.

Now a lot of people think our bodies are alkaline, but when they say that, they are actually referring to our blood which has a slight alkalinity, a pH between 7.35-7.45. Much of our body is actually acidic, and here are some actual numbers:

Tissue	pH	Acidity-Alkalinity
Stomach	1.7 - 3.0	Acidic
Duodenum	5.1 - 6.1	Acidic
Skin	4.5 - 5.5	Acidic
Hair	4.5 - 5.5	Acidic
Vagina	3.5 - 4.9	Acidic
Blood	7.35 - 7.45	Alkaline
Rectum	7 - 8	Alkaline

Now apparently, we have over 75,000 enzymes in our body and enzymes can usually only function in a given pH range. So, it becomes very important that the pH in a given part of the body stays within a given range.

In today's society, due to toxicities, our diet and our water, our bodies are more acidic than we want them to be.

The enzymes required for out gut immune system and the immune systems throughout the body require a given pH to function. The microbiota in our gut, that is both interactive with and supportive of our gut immune system, requires a given pH range in order to live and function.

Yet, the water we drink is not a healthy pH! The water we really want to drink is like that comes off the glaciers and the waterfalls. So further down we will tell how you best create the water our body wants.

Oh, and by the way, did you know that a Dr. Pollock has discovered that the water in the body is not H20 but rather H302 and it is called 'structured water'? There is a reference for his information at the end of the book.

Another quite interesting fact about water is that it has 63 known anomalies. Yeah! There are 63 things about water that don't follow the rules of other compounds or elements. In fact, scientists from around the world are going back to university to research and understand water – it's not what we thought it was!

Of course, apart from the pH of water, we have to look at what is in the water. Actually, pH comes into play here too. The lower the pH of the water the more of those H20 molecules that stick together. For instance, with a pH of 5 – you will get about 18-21 molecules of water sticking together in a formation. Whereas when the pH of water is about 8 – you will only get 3-5 molecules of water sticking together.

So, what does that mean for us? Well the more molecules that stick together, the better the water holds onto or provides a transportation system for all the toxins, heavy metals, pathogens, etc. If the water has a high pH, then it doesn't carry these things into our bodies.

Bottom line, we need to drink good healthy water to support our body functions and immune system. I'll address it further later.

4) By the food we eat

Okay, so we have addressed that our immune system, which we need to protect us from arthritic conditions, can be affected:

- By the air that surrounds us;
- By the air that we breathe; and
- By the water we drink.

I was shocked to learn that there are a huge number of categories of toxins in our foods that our immune system has to deal with.

- Herbicides
- Insecticides
- Pesticides
- Roundup
- Fertilizers
- Artificial colorants
- Stabilizers
- Nitrates/nitrites
- Sugar: both processed and artificial

- Fats: artificial omega 3s, Trans fats, too many omega 6s (they are pro-inflammatory), etc.
- AGEs: advanced glycation Endproducts (see references for further information)

All of these things are unnatural. Our bodies were not designed to deal with them which, in turn, make them toxic to our bodies. Our bodies have to eliminate them, and the gut is predominantly responsible because this is where the food gets metabolized.

All of the above categories can play havoc in our gut by affecting the:

- pH balance;
- Enzymes;
- Immune system; and
- Microbiota.

Which can then leave us susceptible to developing arthritis!

Bottom line, as a society, we need to take care of what we eat, the water, plants and animals. Not just to protect our gut but so that our gut can metabolize the nutrients that the rest of the body requires AND eliminate the pathogens that would do it harm AND support the microbiota that works with the immune system.

Conclusion

Anything and everything that goes into our bodies can affect our immune system! If we want our immune system to protect us and protect us issues that can cause arthritis, we need to protect our immune system.

A simple analogy would be taking care of your car. If you don't care of it, it will fall apart. It needs the oil changed, it needs the water filled, it needs to be cleaned, and it needs fuel in order to run. If anything goes sideways, it starts to falter. If we don't take care of the warning signs, it will eventually just not start.

Be wise, take care of what goes into your body, so that the immune system can take care of you.

Chapter 4

Causes of Inflammation: Toxicity

Toxins form a huge category, it is very overwhelming. But I will keep it simple.

If you have done any research, I am sure you have heard that there are over 75,000 toxic synthetic chemicals that have been introduced into our society since the beginning of the Industrial Revolution.

Some say this number could be 85,000 or 95,000 or even higher. The number keeps going up, so I am not sure exactly how high it is right now, but it is definitely not good.

I often hear people say that 'chemicals' are bad! That is just as misleading as saying the body has an alkaline pH. Just like different parts of the body have a different pH, not all chemicals are bad.

In fact, our bodies are made up of chemicals. The air we breathe or the water we drink or the food we eat is all made up of a huge number of beneficial chemicals. Chemicals are not the problem. The problems arise with the synthetic toxic chemicals!

The toxic chemicals destroy our immune system and it is the toxic chemicals that can provoke arthritic conditions.

The major categories of toxins are:

- Air toxins
- Water toxins
    - What are the added toxins like chloride and fluoride
    - What are the air pollutants
    - What are the ground pollutants
    - What is being released from infrastructure, i.e., copper in the water lines
- Food toxins (there are over 10,000 toxic food additives!!)
    - What the plants breathe
    - What the plants absorb from the soils
    - What is sprayed on the plants
    - What the animals are fed
    - What the animals are injected with
    - Added colorants
    - Added preservatives for shelf life
    - Added artificial flavorings
    - Added synthetic vitamins, minerals, omega 3s

o Heavy metals, i.e., mercury in fish; arsenic in chicken

o SUGAR is a huge toxin to the body!!! We will explore that at the end of the chapter. Here are 12 categories that you really need to avoid, according to the Environmental Working Group (EWG)[4]:

1. Nitrites and nitrates (carcinogenic)
2. Potassium bromate (carcinogenic)
3. Propyl paraben (endocrine disrupters)
4. Butylated hydroxy anisole (BHA) (carcinogenic)
5. Butylated hydroxytoluene (BHT) (carcinogenic)
6. Propyl gallate (endocrine disrupters, carcinogenic)
7. Theobromine (can cause headaches)
8. Secret flavor ingredients
9. Artificial colors (cancer, nerve damage)
10. Diacetyl (Alzheimer's & cancer)
11. Phosphate-based food additives (Watch List)
12. Aluminum-based additives (Watch List)

- Cleaning product toxins
- Hygiene product toxins
- Makeup product toxins

- o Note there are a number of companies who claim that there are no alcohols, parabens, etc. when in fact there are.
- Household cleaner product toxins
- Clothing product toxins

Wow! That includes virtually all of life. And I am not going to list all the toxins in each category. But a really good site to explore if you are interested in the different toxins is EWG.org – they list the toxins in a wide variety of ways, alphabetically, categorically, by product, even by given product label. For instance, if you wanted to identify the toxins in a given brand of makeup, you could just type into your browser: EWG, product name, specific product item and you will probably get what you are looking for.

Wait a minute, there is a huge amount of toxins in another entirely separate category – electromagnetic frequencies or waves – that can cause havoc to our systems and actually throw the immune system into chaos. In fact, one article published in *Pathophysiology* and referenced on PubMed states that, "EMFs disturb immune function through stimulation of various allergic and inflammatory responses, as well as effects on tissue repair processes. Such disturbances increase the risks for various diseases including cancer.[5]

Now remember, I said I would come back to sugar. Well excess sugar in the body turns into AGEs (Advanced Glycation Endproducts). There are apparently over 100 of them AND they are incredibly toxic to the body. They attach to cells anywhere in the body. In the gut, in the blood vessels, in the brain, in the organs, ANYWHERE!!! They cause the cells to dysfunction, provoke cancer, or the cells can die. This is huge. Have you any idea how many foods have sugar, high fructose corn syrup, beet sugar, and all the artificial sugars? They all cause damage to the body!!!

So, as you can see, we are surrounded by and ingesting toxins, and we need to be aware and proactive about avoiding them. The immune system and the liver have the primary responsibility of getting rid of them. In fact, a really important compound to both the immune system and the liver is glutathione. But we will get to that later.

Is it any wonder that the immune system can get overwhelmed and confused and start to:

- Create allergies to things we don't need to be allergic to;
- Think that our body is the pathogen;
- Fail to resolve inflammation – the inflammatory system is a part of the immune system; or

- Fail to protect us from pathogens?

Unfortunately, any of these things can lead to arthritic conditions.

Bottom line is, we are loaded with toxins from all sides. Those toxins can accumulate in the body, disrupt body functions, and, in the end, can cause arthritic conditions. We need to be careful. Modern society creates a painful way of dying.

And all Western Conventional Medicine can do for us is hand us toxic prescriptions.

Chapter 5

Causes of Inflammation: Trauma

Trauma is identified as any kind of physical impact on the body that tears, breaks or otherwise damages the body, and in particular, bones, cartilage, ligaments, tendons, synovial fluid bags (found between connecting bones), meniscus.

Now the body has all kinds of healing processes. It goes through the massive inflammatory process where messengers (cytokines) are sent throughout the body to warn of the damage and to bring in all the different crews, both local and generalized, to work on the healing.

Then there are the anti-inflammatory processes that involve a variety of stages in healing and getting rid of the debris and by-products provoked by the healing processes.

But there are few predominant issues that can happen here.

1) If the inflammation doesn't heal effectively, we are left with a subclinical inflammation with no

overt symptoms, that can cause a number of compromised functions throughout life which have a domino effect.

2) If the required nutrients are not available during the healing process and/or the body is not given the time to heal effectively and we end up with either fibrosis or other conditions that ultimately cause a domino effect (see below for more on fibrosis).

3) Fibrosis can also occur when the body heals too fast causing excess fibers or connective tissue. When you see a scar on a person, that can also be the result of healing too fast. So, think of fibrosis as being internal scarring, from healing too fast.

4) Toxins, heavy metals, AGEs, etc. get caught up in the healing process and prevent effective processes from occurring which end up having a domino effect.

Now I mentioned fibrosis with number two and three. When our bodies are growing and building initially, all the connective tissues grow in nice straight lines. But when fibrosis happens, the lines get all disorganized. So, a simple analogy would be to hold your hands out with your fingers stretched out straight – that is how the connective usually starts. Now cross your fingers over on another and twist your hands, which is what fibrosis might look like. A simple analogy, but it works for our purposes here.

Any of these conditions, or any combination of them, and probably ones I have no idea about, can all cause arthritic conditions down the road.

Bottom line, if you have an accident, make sure you provide the body with the nutrients it needs to heal, as opposed to the drugs, and give it time to heal properly – or there will be consequences.

Chapter 6

Causes of Inflammation: Prescription Drugs

Now this is a nasty one, but we have to deal with it. Yes, drugs can cause arthritic conditions.

- Did you know that most drugs deplete the body of nutrients?
- Did you know that half of the most commonly prescribed drugs cause cancer?
- Did you know that drugs have lubricants in them to protect the machinery that makes them – that can be very toxic to the body AND can prevent the body from absorbing the active ingredient?
- Did you know that statin drugs can cause muscle inflammation & pain?
- Did you know that more than 80 drugs can cause Lupus (SLE) that looks like rheumatoid arthritis?[6,7]

There are many other kinds of problems with prescription drugs:

- Physicians are told about the relative risk NOT the absolute risk. Relative risk refers to when the numbers drop from 3 to 2 out of 1000. The drop from 3 to 2 is a relative drop of 30% or relative risk. On the other hand, absolute risk is referring to the fact that it has dropped from 3/1000 to 2/1000 which the drop of 0.002% which is absolute risk. In fact, when physicians are told the truth about a given prescription, prescriptions drop significantly – which is why Big Pharma doesn't tell them.
- Physicians are taught about the safety, efficacy other factors regarding the particular drug, but only what the Pharmaceutical company wants them to know.
  - Recently I had a discussion with a physician who prescribed a drug for a friend of mine. I phoned to talk with the MD claiming I was very concerned about the drug. She attempted to convince me that the drug was safe and effective. After all, she had just been to the Pharmaceutical Conference that explained how safe their new drug was. I couldn't believe the MD was that naïve. Of course, the pharmaceutical company was only going to tell them about the positives. I had to give the MD the legal site that already had three class action law suits against the drug/Pharmaceutical company!

- Did you know that Big Pharma pays for the lawyers and judges for the FDA?[3]
- Did you know that Big Pharma controls the curriculum for most medical schools?
- Did you know that Big Pharma controls the protocol and procedure that MDs have to follow – or be sued, fined or lose their license to practice?
- Did you know that Big Pharma actually represents a huge part of the US Federal Government? There are 30 members of the Federal Government who are also representing pharmaceutical companies and Monsanto.

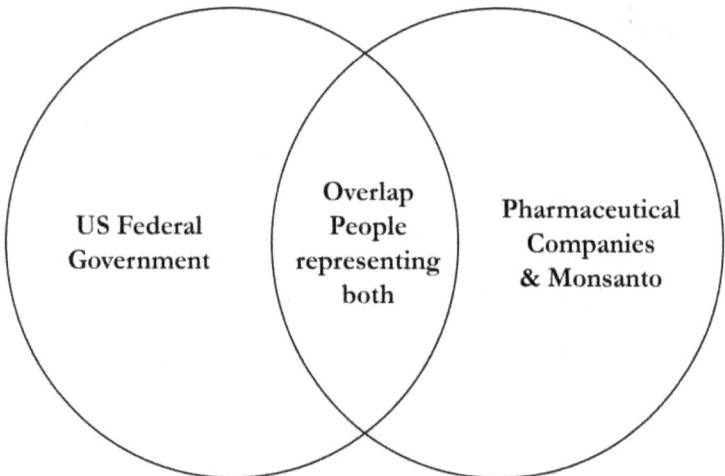

US Federal Government | Overlap People representing both | Pharmaceutical Companies & Monsanto

- As you can see, there is an overlap between Monsanto/Big Pharma and the Federal Government.

- Did you know that if you combine the deaths caused by MDs, hospitals and pharmaceutical drugs – you now have the number one cause of death?[8]

One article that is very worth reading is "Death by Medicine", it is listed in the references.

There are a few things you can do when you are given a prescription to take:

1) Do a Google search and type in the name of the prescription and type in "law suits" after it.
2) Also, type in the name of the prescription and type in "side effects" after it.

If you determine that you do not want to take the prescriptions due to either the lawsuits and/or the side-effects, you may want to take your research into your family physician and ask him for an alternative, or go to a REAL health practitioner and ask them what they would suggest.

Bottom line is, do your due diligence. It is your body! MDs are being scammed by Big Pharma just as much as we are. Unfortunately, very few do their due diligence, so it up to us to protect our bodies.

Chapter 7

Causes of Inflammation: Dehydration

Now dehydration is another funny one.

We are constantly being told to drink more water. Why? Because of the old belief that you should drink 8, 8 oz glasses of water a day. Right?

Did you know that the woman that wrote the article back in 1968, about dehydration and drinking 8, 8 oz of glasses of water was interviewed? She was shocked at how her "suggestion" became the '8x8' rule overnight! There was never any science behind it. She had suggested as something to do when you had a major workout and had lost a lot of fluid in your sweat!

Unbelievable!

Even naturopathic colleges preach this 8x8 rule! Yes, your body requires water. Yes, we are told that we are about 70% water. But the body tells you when you are thirsty, just like it tells you when you are hungry.

Further, if you remember earlier in this book, I told you about Dr Pollock's work and how he claims that we really don't have a lot of H20 in the body, but rather H302. H302 is called "Structured Water". And it makes sense that the body can best turn H20 into H302 when it is given good clean high pH water – remember that means fewer H20 molecules clustered together.

How much water do you think there is in fruit and vegetables compared to your body? If we were eating healthy fruits and vegetables, we would be getting a lot of our water from them, I would think. Even meat has water in it. Well as long you don't cook it and then cook it again – which is one of the many reasons that 'medium rare' apparently has more nutrients for the body than meat that is 'well done'.

Anyways, whether you abide by a more vegetarian diet or a more paleo diet, your diet should include a lot of fruit and vegetables that have a lot of water in them.

Now, the flip side of the coin with water is you can get too much! Actual research shows that an excess of water can:

- Cause problems with your blood vessels;
- Cause problems with your kidneys;

- Which in turn can cause problems with your heart;
- Can throw off several functions in the body if it is too acidic; and
- If the water has a low pH, it creates huge molecular structures that carry even more toxins into your body

But let's look at why water is important to the joints and arthritis. Most of the connective tissues, like bones and muscles, do have water in them. And in particular, your synovial fluid cavities. These cavities are like a bag full of a particular kind of fluid that allows the bones to move back and forth without rubbing against one another. In a sense they act like shock absorbers.

Well, if any of these connective tissues or the synovial fluid cavities get dehydrated, they are going to shrink. Think about it, virtually anything else in nature will shrink when it loses water. Think of a plant that has "dried" up.

Now if the connective tissue dries up there is no protection from one bone rubbing against the other – and voila, you have an arthritic condition.

What is the bottom line here? Drink healthy water. Drink water when your body tells you to! You eat when you are hungry. So, drink water when you are thirsty! Not because some cosmopolitan magazine suggested it. But make sure you drink healthy water.

Go to Chapter 13 and learn how to create your own healthy water.

Chapter 8

Causes of Inflammation: Auto-immune Disease

I really enjoyed understanding auto-immune disease. I thought it was a fascinating topic. Unfortunately, like so many other issues, it can also be really complex. Actually, the whole immune system is an incredibly complex system. But I promise I will do my best to explain it in simple Grandma terms.

The immune system protects you from harm. It is made up of:

- The innate system: is derived from elements we are born with or given to us by our mother during delivery or in breast milk; and
- The adaptive system: learns as it grows and reacts to pathogens.

Apparently, the red bone marrow not only makes the red blood cells that pick-up oxygen from the lungs and delivers it through the body. Along the way, these red blood cells pick up CO_2 and take the

C02 back to the lungs so the lungs can expel it. The bone marrow also makes leukocytes which identify and remember enemy pathogens and helps the body destroy them. There are a variety of leukocytes.

- Phagocytes: eat up the pathogens – there are 3 types
  o Neutrophils: eat up bacteria
  o Eosinophils: fight parasites and deal with allergic reactions
  o Monocytes: big eaters that eat enemy cells and produce cytokines
- Basophils: deal with allergies and inflammation
  o Lymphocytes: B & T cells and they start the reaction against pathogens

So, what happens with auto-immune disorders? In a variety of different situations, the immune system can get confused. The immune system starts to think that the body itself, or some part of the body, is the pathogen or the invader. And so, it does what it is supposed to do with any invader. It destroys it. That is what the immune system is supposed to.

But obviously, the immune system is destroying the wrong thing. The immune system has turned on itself. That is the simple version of what ends up happening.

Now we have to find a simple understanding of how that can possibly happen when the body is wise and so beautifully designed.

The following is a simple list of what might happen if our immune system is compromised.

1) Low Glutathione

Insufficient nutrients and/or an overwhelming amount of toxins and/or an upheaval in our hormones can cause low levels of glutathione.

Yes, the word is glue/ta/thigh/on. Big word. But then that compound does more things in the body that almost any other compound in the body.

It is made in every cell of the body, although the highest concentrations are found in the liver and the brain.

It is often only thought of as the Master Anti-oxidant – which is huge in and of itself, but it does a lot more than that.

- First, let's look at why it is called the Master Anti-oxidant.
  a) It is an anti-oxidant, and like other anti-oxidants it eliminates free radicals.
  b) All other anti-oxidants only work on one type of free radical – glutathione works on all categories of free radicals.

c) All other anti-oxidants only work in one area of the body, for instance, in the cell; the cell membrane; or outside of the cell – whereas glutathione works everywhere.

d) All other anti-oxidants can only function as an anti-oxidant once, and then becomes free radical that the body has to eliminate – usually a much easier free radical that the type it was eliminating.

   i. Glutathione on the other not only re-stabilizes itself so that it can function over and over and over again.

   ii. But it also re-stabilizes all kinds of other anti-oxidants so they can function again.

- But it doesn't just address free radicals, it is also the body's primary chelator – which means that it eliminates heavy metals from the body which is important because heavy metals can do a lot of damage to the body and deplete the body of vital nutrients.

- It is also a major component of each cell's detoxification system.

- It is also a major component of the liver's detoxification system – which is one of the reasons why the highest concentration is found in the liver. The liver has several detox systems which involve two, three or four phases. Usually at the final stage a glutathione compound is added and then the reformed compound is delivered back into the intestines to be eliminated.

- It is the only known compound in the body that protects the mitochondria. Every cell has a multitude of mitochondria that produce the fuel for everything that happens in a given cell.
- It regulates the nitric oxide (NO)in the body – which is involved in the immune system and other functions like vasodilation (the relaxation of blood vessels) and hormone regulation.
- It is involved either directly or indirectly (through compounds like nitric oxide – that it regulates) in the regulations of all the hormones in the body.
- It is involved in the regulation of calcium movement in the body, especially in heart cells.
- It is the only known compound, so far, that not only protects the telomeres (compounds at the end of the DNA that are required for replication) but actually promotes the enzyme telomerase to make new telomeres – which is huge in anti-aging.
- It protects DNA from becoming dysfunctional.
- It is involved in protein synthesis in the cells.
- It is required to transport amino acids around inside of our cells.
- It is required in red blood cells, so that they can both pick up/drop off both oxygen and CO_2.

- Now if that were not enough for one little compound, it is hugely important in the immune system! How? Well let me tell you:
  a) It is required for immune cells to develop, like the ones I mentioned before: T cells and B cells, macrophages, and other ones like: tumor necrosis factor (TNF), natural killer cells (NK), etc.
  b) It is required for immune cells to react/respond.
  c) It is required to keep a healthy balance between different types of immune cells, for instance, T1 and T2 cells. If either is more dominant, we are susceptible to a number of disorders including auto-immune disorders.
- And finally, we need to look at its role in inflammation, which of course is a big part of any arthritic condition.
  a) When the pro-inflammatory processes start, Nitric Oxide is used to relax the membrane (smooth muscles) of the blood vessels to allow all kinds of compounds to move in and out of the damaged site – remember I told you that glutathione regulates Nitric Oxide.
  b) Both the pro-inflammatory and the anti-inflammatory processes in the body produce a lot of free radicals – which cause oxidative stress – which causes inflammation – so

glutathione is required to eliminate the free radicals (other compounds in the body do this as well, but glutathione is by far the most important).

c) Glutathione is required by the red blood cells that bring oxygen to the area and take away the excess CO_2 that occurs with inflammation.

d) Glutathione is required by the white blood cells both to develop and respond to the damaged area that occurs with inflammation.

e) Glutathione is required by all the cells to protect the mitochondria that produce the fuel for the healing process, and of course even more is required when there is inflammation.

f) Glutathione is required to transport amino acids around the cells so that the cells can make all the products required to repair the damage that occurs with inflammation.

All in all, glutathione ends up being a big part of the healing process. AND, if there is insufficient glutathione, then the repair doesn't happen, or it happens ineffectively. When the inflammation or damage is not repaired properly, guess what we get? You guessed it! Arthritis!

Now can you imagine one little compound being responsible for all of that? I was amazed.

But then I started to look at all the different things that can decrease or destroy our glutathione levels and I was even more amazed.

- Aging
- Dehydration
- Exercising past a sweat
- Food additives
- Genetic abnormalities
- Herbicides
- Infections
- Injuries
- Insecticides
- Lack of nutrients
- Pesticides
- Pollution
- Poor sleeping habits
- Prescription drugs and illegal drugs
- Radiation and chemotherapy
- Stress (and who doesn't have that – either in the psyche or in the gut)
- Sunburns

WOW! And that's the short list! So, I thought, I will go the health food store and buy some of that glutathione – which they do sell. But then the practitioners at the Gibson's Clinic told me that the hydrochloric acid in the stomach, which breaks down all the proteins that we eat, will break down the glutathione compound and when that happens, then we tend to lose one of the amino acids, specifically the cysteine.

So, then I thought, they say that as we get older, we make less of that hydrochloric acid – so then maybe I wouldn't break down the glutathione? But apparently, even if I didn't break it down in the stomach, the compound is way too big to get into a cell anyways. So, the cells do have to make it.

Well okay then. My next question was: what do the cells need to make glutathione? Well this is where it can get really complicated – but I will try to explain in Grandma terms.

It takes three major components, in every cell, that have to function properly, in order to regulate (like anything else, you don't want too much) and make glutathione.

- The mitochondria need to be making fuel.
- The DNA need to be making the proper mRNA & other RNA tools.
- The Methylation Cycle needs to have 4 components functioning:
  - The methionine cycle;
  - The folate cycle;
  - The biopterin cycle; and
  - The urea cycle.

Now there is no way, this old Grandma is going to go and try to explain all that to you. But I thought I would give you the terms so that if you wanted to look any of them up you could.

The bottom line: you need healthy cells to regulate and create glutathione. By the way, in Chapter 12 there is a list of the foods that support the functioning of the cell components I listed.

2) Dysfunctional Immune System

One cause can be the immune system itself is dysfunctional. This can be due to:

- AGEs (Advanced Glycation Endproducts);
- Environmental toxins;
- Excess free radicals;
- Heavy metals;
- Excessive or chronic stress (psychologically or in the gut);
- Sugars.

So how do these different things cause damage to the immune system? Well they all can interrupt the cellular processes in different ways. For instance, AGEs attach to the cells and cause disruption in both the cell membrane and what goes in and out of the cell, not only with the immune system cells but with all cells in the body.

Free radicals run around stealing electrons from other molecules and cause dysfunction, oxidative stress and ultimately inflammation, not only in the immune system but anywhere in the body.

Processed sugars are toxic to the body and the brain and can cause disruption in a number of different ways, again in the immune system and everywhere else in the body. Despite the fact that there are a huge number of causes of cancer and a wide variety of cancers, in general, cancer cells require 4 to 10 times the amount of sugar to function compared to a regular cell. Now remember, this is Grandma talking and I recognize this is very simplified.

Now, Grandma here used to think that I could just use the artificial sugars and that was okay. Boy did I find out otherwise. They are just as bad as the table sugars and some are even worse! A tip that I found out from the Gibsons was that if I really needed to sweeten something up, I should use either unpasteurized honey or Stevia. So that is all I use now.

Heavy metals and other toxins can cause plaque along the arteries, disrupt neural functioning, interrupt neurotransmitter function, get caught in the mucosal lining – whether it be in the gut; in the respiratory tract (nose, throat, lungs), or in the reproductive tracts (penile and vaginal mucosa) – or even destroy the microbiota in the gut.

The Gibsons explained to me all the common places that you can get heavy metal toxins from.

- Aluminum: aluminum cookware, antiperspirant, contaminated water, over the counter drugs, several douche brands, some baking powders, various refined foods (flour, baking goods, processed cheeses, table salt).
- Arsenic: chicken, contaminated water, cotton plants, pesticides.
- Cadmium: cigarette smoke, contaminated water, fish, plants.
- Lead: contaminated water, glass, lead batteries, leaded gasoline, paint, rubber products.
- Mercury: tooth fillings, vaccinations, salmon (the larger the fish, the more there is due to larger fish feeding on smaller ones).

3) Imbalanced Gut Bacteria

The mutual inter-dynamic relationship between the immune system and the gut bacteria and other gut microbes is complex. So, if the microbiota becomes dysfunctional – so can the immune system and vice versa.

We have over 35,000 possible species of good bacteria in the gut along with various virus, molds, yeast, etc. According to Wikipedia, microbiota means "the ecological community of commensal, symbiotic and pathogenic microorganisms that literally share our body space."[9]

Apparently most of our gut bacteria comes from between 30-40 species of bacteria. The fascinating thing here, is that we have more bacteria in our gut than cells in our whole body!

That means that there is more that is not us than is us. I love that. And here we thought we were so important in our own bodies. How arrogant we are. Did you know that the gut bacteria, the microbiota, can affect your thoughts, your emotions and your behavior? Wow, that's scary. Good reason to keep the good healthy ones strong.

4) Infection that the immune system can't handle effectively

Now the interesting thing here is that the evidence shows that we if have a healthy immune system, a bad pathogen cannot survive. They can only survive if we have a weakened immune system and/or an imbalance in our gut bacteria. Why both? Because they go hand in hand – remember they work interactively.

So, whether our immune system is weak, or we have an imbalance or a depleted microbiota, then we are more susceptible to both infections and inflammation (in the gut and elsewhere) that can even further weaken the system. And make us more susceptible to arthritis!

Let's look at some of the infections that may be more related to arthritic conditions.

- Lyme disease depletes the body of oxygen and is associated with:
  o Arthritis
  o Heart muscle disruption
  o Neurological abnormalities
  o And other issues.
- Rheumatoid arthritis can affect:
  o Joints
  o Heart & blood vessels
  o Kidneys
  o Lungs
  o Skin
- Septicemia caused by:
  o Bacteria
    - Staphylococcus aureus
    - Hemophilus influenza
    - E. coli
    - Pseudomonas spp.
    - Neisseria gonorrhoeae
    - Salmonella spp.
    - Mycobacterium tuberculosis
  o Viral
    - Hepatitis A, B and C

71

- Parvovirus B19
- Herpes
- HIV
- AIDS
- HTLV-1
- Adenovirus
- Coxsackie
- Mumps
- Ebola
- Fungi
  - Histoplasma
  - Coccidioides
  - Blastomyces

Any of these pathogenic organisms can cause arthritic conditions, either by hiding out in our joints and causing problems or by directly compromising our immune system which then impacts on our joints.

5) Pathogens in your teeth

Yes, your teeth and gums can be the source of an auto-immune disease.

Now you have to read this. It is fascinating. Have you ever heard of a Dr. Weston Price? He was a dentist and a scientist that worked around the world and in conjunction with the Mayo Clinic. The research team had six PhDs and a microbiologist who identified the bacteria.

The bacteria in the teeth and gums, and as far away from a given tooth as 1.5 inches, were shown to cause everything from congestive heart failure to Auto Immune diseases to DNA alterations!!!

One group of bacteria are called "porins". They drill holes in the red blood cells which allows the hemoglobin to leak into the surrounding blood where the bacteria 'suck' up the iron!!

Hey, that iron is there for us – not you guys!!

Apparently, his work was intentionally buried, and dentists were not taught a lot of what Dr. Weston discovered with regard to:

- Amalgams;
- Nickel crowns;
- Pathogens in teeth; and
- Root canals.

He identified the tubules for each tooth (one tooth may have upwards of 80 tubules in the dentin) and where these tubules went to in the body, how the pathogens traveled through the body, and the damage that they could cause!

Would you believe that most dentists don't know any of this material!! You may want to read this very interesting article about root canals.[10]

Other pathogens associated with the teeth are:

- Capnocytophaga ochnacea
- Fungi
- Gemella morbillorum
- Klebsiella oxytoca
- Neisseria meningitidis
  - Pseudomonas aeruginosa
  - Meningitis
  - Spirochetes
  - Staphylococcus family
  - Streptococcus family
  - And more

Do you think this might be a good reason to make sure that your teeth are kept in good health? I put the references at the back of the book for you, but you can quickly go to drwestonprice.com for more information.

Chapter 9

Pain Killers – Watch Out

Now virtually anyone who has suffered from arthritis has asked for pain killers. Whether they are OTCs, prescriptions, natural, or whatever. It is difficult to live with that ongoing pain all day long.

I know it was difficult for me. I don't know whether my pain threshold is low, medium or high, and quite frankly I don't care. Pain is horrible and when you get no relief – it can destroy your life. I don't know about you, but I can sure understand why some people can get hooked on illegal drugs in an attempt to deal with their pain. Simply because the MD handed out the prescription, I wasn't considered a criminal user, but I was sure addicted to the prescription drugs. I couldn't make it through a day without taking pain killers my physician prescribed for me.

I never thought of myself as being addicted until I started doing the research on the prescriptions and how they are all addictive. I learned how the drugs affect the physiological functioning as well as the neurological functioning. That really scared me. Many of the prescriptive pain killers are also highly associated with suicidal behavior. Holy cow!

My doctor never told me any of that. I was shocked. I knew that I couldn't function even minimally during the day without the drugs and I couldn't sleep without the drugs, but I just never thought of myself as an addict.

Thankfully, I had the guidance of the health practitioners at the Gibson Clinic. They not only helped me to wean off the the prescriptions, but also to eliminate the arthritis. If this is a concern for you, make sure you find good health practitioners to help you wean off the prescription drugs because they are dangerous and you cannot just stop taking them.

Both pain and pain killers can destroy our lives and our relationships. Living with pain is exhausting both physically and emotionally which in turn permeates through every part of our life.

So, what do we do? We want to stop the pain so we look for pain killers.

But when we really start to look at the prescription medications – we can get pretty scared. Here are a few issues and then a few examples.

Issues

- The pain killers never solve the underlying problem.
- Many times, the meds don't even cover up the pain.
- Many of the pain killers are addictive, no better than street drugs.
- Most, if not all, pain killers can cause a huge number of other dangerous issues:
  o Stomach issues,
  o Small intestine issues,
  o Liver issues,
  o Addiction, and
  o Nutrient depletion.

That's just the short list of problems they can cause. When I started to read this stuff, I got really scared. So, I did some further research.

Let's look at some examples

1) Cox 2 inhibitors: Celebrex, Celecoxib

   i.   They can triple the risk of a heart attack – it's even on the box.
   ii.   They cause gastrointestinal problems.

2) NSAIDs – that stands for Nonsteroidal anti-inflammatory drugs: Advil, Aleve, Ibuprofen, Naproxen

i. Over 16,000 die a year from NSAIDs in the US alone[11]
ii. Biggest cause of gastrointestinal bleeding
iii. Biggest cause of gut ulcers

3) Opiates – Percocet's/dan, Hydrocodone, Oxycodone, Vicodin, Lorcet, Norco

i. Over 37,000 a year die from prescribed Opiates in the US alone. The numbers went from about 37,000 in 2006[12] to over 72,000 in 2017!![13]
ii. They are very addictive
iii. They can cause ruptured bowels
iv. They can cause respiratory dysfunction
v. They can cause coma
vi. They can cause a cardiac arrest
vii. They also cause depression

4) Tylenol, acetaminophen

i. Over 50,000 land in the emergency award a year, in the US alone from overuse
ii. Liver toxicity
iii. Nausea
iv. Abdominal pain
v. Bleeding/bruising

5) Aspirin, acetylsalicylates (which is the synthetic form of a compound found in willow bark)

i. Causes intestinal bleeding

    ii.   Causes perforated ulcers

    iii.   Causes Reyes Syndrome in children and young adults (about 95% of Reyes Syndrome is due to using aspirin)

6) Corticosteroids (powerful anti-inflammatory drugs used for Rheumatoid arthritis to suppress an overactive immune system)

    i.   More likely to get infections

    ii.   Higher blood sugars

    iii.   Bone thinning

Kind of scary isn't it? And that was just the short list.

Bottom line: get rid of the underlying problem and try something else for the pain in the short term.

Chapter 10

Foods for Arthritis

Why should we buy anti-inflammatories when we can get them in our food? Do we really have that much of an obligation to support Big Pharma? Do we really have that much money to waste?

Now you might feel that pills are the easy way to go – no responsibility to your health and don't have to look after your diet. But you will end up suffering even more if you go that route. But then, the choice is yours.

Now, if you are like me and fed up taking all those pills and would really like a healthier way to go and want to eliminate the inflammation, then stick with me and keep reading.

Omega 3s

First off, did you know that even the American Surgeon General recommended cod liver oil? Yeah, that horrible stuff our mothers and grandmothers used to make us take! Well the nice thing about it today is, you can get it in pills.

Cod Liver Oil not only has the anti-inflammatory omega 3s in it, but it also has Vitamin A and Vitamin D, both of which are important to repair cartilage damage, which it has been shown to do. Wow, that's sounds pretty good doesn't it?

Now I am sure that you have heard that Omega 3s are good for you but did you know that they are anti-inflammatories?

Omega 3 is a fatty acid and all fatty acids have the same basic chemical structure. There are a huge number of different types of fatty acids and they are organized in numbered categories, for instance omega 3s, omega 6s and omega 9s. The 3s, 6s and the 9s refer to where there is a double bond between the carbon compounds, which I am not going to get into further here.

What we need to know is that the omega 3 group of fatty acids are anti-inflammatory, and the omega 6 group of fatty acids are pro-inflammatory. So obviously it becomes really important to eat foods that are high in omega 3 and low in omega 6.

Now apparently even in each group there are a number of different types of fatty acids depending on the additional chemical structures. And Grandma here doesn't want to get into all of that. But I did think you should understand the basic differences.

So, let's look at some foods with good fatty acids.

Foods to work with

General rule of thumb, foods that are:

- Whole foods
- Organic foods
- 30% of the diet should be raw foods

Fish

- Anchovy
- Herring
- Mackerel
- Salmon – we need to be careful of farmed salmon
- Sardines
- Whitefish

Fruit

- 100% Chocolate (see below for more information)
- Avocados

Oils

- Avocado oil
- Coconut oil
- Fish oil
- Flax seed oil

- Hemp oil
- Olive oil – most olive oil today has lost its omega 3s and so it has to be added back in and usually synthetic, so it is best to avoid it.

Seeds

- Flax seed – make sure that it is ground
- Hemp seed
- Salba seed/Chia seed

Spices

- Dried marjoram
- Dried oregano
- Fresh basil
- Ground cloves

Vegetables

- Chinese broccoli
- Frozen spinach

Foods to Avoid

Based on how they are grown

- Foods sprayed with:
  o Herbicides
  o Insecticides
  o Pesticides
  o POPs (Persistent Organic Pollutants)

- GMO foods

Based on how they are processed

- Fast foods
- Microwaved foods
- Pasteurized foods
- Processed foods

Inflammatory foods

- Allergen foods, like nightshade vegetables
  – especially if you have Rheumatoid
  Arthritis
  o Eggplant
  o Peppers
  o Potatoes
  o Tomatoes
- Dairy
- Grains/flours (typically sprayed with
  Roundup – a known carcinogen)
- Oxalic acid foods:
  o Cranberries
  o Plum
  o Rhubarb
  o Spinach
- Red meat (can provoke gout which is in
  the arthritic family)
- Seeds and oils that are high in Omega 6s:

- o Corn oil (note that we cannot digest corn unless it is popped)
  - o Safflower oil
  - o Soybean oil
  - o Sunflower seeds/oil
- Shellfish
- Simple carbohydrates, they turn to sugar quickly and exaggerate the pain
- Sugar
- Other products:
  - o Alcohol
  - o Coffee
  - o Table sat – use mineral salts
  - o Tobacco

Before moving on, here are some simple rules that the Gibsons share:

1) Don't drink water with meals – dilutes the enzymes.
   a. Drink water before a meal – it helps to fill you up.
2) Avoid the whites: dairy, flour, potatoes, rice and sugar.
   a. White rice is better than brown rice which holds the toxins.
3) Eat fruits on an empty stomach – they get digested better that way.
4) Eat good healthy fats – they are anti-inflammatory.

5) Eat good healthy mineral salts and bathe in Epsom salts.

Chapter 11

Herbs for Arthritis

According to the Gibsons, the herbs are incredibly powerful. But they have to be taken in the right combination and the right dosage because they are so powerful.

The Gibsons always laugh and say:

"When Conventional Medicine wants to negate us, they say that 'foods and herbs have no proven impact'; but then they turn around and say that 'foods and herbs can interfere with their synthetic drugs' and of course, 'they like to blame us if something goes wrong'. How can both be right?

AND, they forget that so many of the drugs are simply artificial synthetic replications of the compounds found in those foods and herbs. Unfortunately, the compound has been isolated from all the other compounds that it works with AND is now synthetic. But it is expected to have the same impact!

Unfortunately, the impact of a whole compound found in its natural environment is very different from an isolated synthetic compound. Further, they end up depleting the body of nutrients and causing other problems."

But let's get back on track here. Here is a list of the precautions with herbs that the Gibsons provide.

Herbal Precautions

1) Herbs are powerful – they must be taken in the right dosage and right combination or they can cause additional issues.
2) Herbs can interact with your medication – ask your herbalist, Dr. of Natural Medicine or Naturopath – they usually have a lot more information than your MD. Many of the REAL health practitioner programs include a comprehensive study of Western Conventional Medicine. The MDs have only studied their side, and as you learned earlier from the Editor-in-Chiefs of two of the most prestigious journals, they can't be trusted – they are typically up to 40 years behind AND are taught by Big Pharma.

So, let's provide a simple example. If you are already on a drug that is meant to bring down high blood pressure and now you also take an herb (or a combination of herbs, dietary protocols and/or supplements) that is also meant to bring down high blood pressure, your blood pressure may go too low.

3) On the other hand, a given herb or supplement may interfere with a given drugs. For instance, if you are taking a chemotherapy that works by destroying the glutathione in your body and you take herbs or supplements that help you increase glutathione in your body (because you want to strengthen your own immune system – which makes sense); then you are going to interfere with how the chemotherapy functions in your body. Personally, I would go for enabling my body to do the work rather than disabling it. But that's Grandma for you.

4) You need to be consistent and follow the instructions given to you.

5) You need to know when to take them, for instance, before or after surgery, with or without food, in the morning or in the evening, etc.

6) You need to be able to know what to take. For instance, you don't take an immune enhancing herb if the immune system is already overactive.

7) You need to know which of the species is most helpful. For instance, there are a huge number of species but only a few types of red reishi have been studied! The two most studies are: Ganoderma lucidum and G.sinensis. The G.lucidum is commonly called Red Reishi. It is the one most commonly used in herbal medicine for inflammation.

8) When you work with herbs, you need to know what part of the plant that you need to work with. For instance, it may be the root or the leaf or the bark or the berry. Each have different nutrient profiles. The easiest part to grow and harvest will obviously be the cheapest to purchase, but may not be what you need.

Sounds like a good reason to see someone who really knows what they are talking about. At the Gibson's Clinic, Pappy is a Master Herbalist and he knows his herbs inside and out.

The following is a short list of herbs that have a great impact on arthritic conditions – if taken properly. The first name is the common name, the name in brackets is the Latin name, and the second set of brackets identifies some of the compounds that are considered to be the 'active ingredient'. Just don't forget that the 'active ingredient' works best when it is still working in conjunction with all of the other compounds in that plant.

Common Kitchen Herbs for Inflammation

- Basil *(Ocimum basilicum)* (polyphenolic flavonoids)
- Black pepper *(Piper nigrum)* (pepperine)
- Cardamom *(Elettaria cardamomum)* (compound 1,8-cineole)
- Cilantro *(Coriandrum sativum)* (quercetin)
- Cinnamon *(Cinnamomum verum)* (phenolic, triterpenoids)
- Cloves *(Syzgium aromaticum)* (eugenol)
- Fennel seeds *(Foeniculum vulgare)* (anethole)
- Garlic *(Allium sativum)* (sulfur containing compounds, allin)
- Ginger *(Zingiber off)* (curcuminiods)
- Oregano *(Origanum vulgare)* (phenols)
- Rosemary *(Rosmarinus off.)* (carnosol)
- Sage *(Salvia off.)* (flavones, phenolic, triterpenoids)
- Turmeric *(Curcuma longa)* (curcumin)

When you get these herbs from an Herbalist, they will give them to you in tincture form which is much stronger than anything you will get in the kitchen.

Herbs for Pain

- Arnica *(Arnica montana)* (sesquiterpene lactones)
- Boswellia *(4 types used for arthritis)* (Incensole Acetate)
- Devils claw *(Harpagophytum procumbens)* (iridoid glycosides)
- Ginger *(Zingiber off)* (curcuminiods)
- Turmeric *(Curcuma longa)* (curcumin)
- Willow bark *(Salix alba)* (Salicylic acid)
- Yarrow *(Achillea millefolium)* (Triterpene, flavinoids)

Herbs for Rheumatoid Arthritis

- Boswellia *(4 types used for arthritis)* (Incensole Acetate)
- Ginger *(Zingiber off)* (curcuminiods)
- Green tea *(Camellia sinensis)* (polyphenols EGCG)
- Turmeric *(Curcuma longa)* (curcumin)
- White willow bark *(Salix)* (salicin)

Herbs to Support the Immune System

- Astragalus *(Astragalus membranaceus)* (polysaccharides, saponins)
- Echinacea (especially *E.augustofolia*) (alkamides)

- Garlic *(Allium sativum)* (sulfur containing compounds, allin)
- Ginger *(Zingiber off)* (curcuminiods)
- Ginseng (all the different types but especially Siberian & Ashwagandha)
- Stinging Nettles (*Urtica diocia*) (polysaccharides)

Herbs that Help to Restore Health to the Gut

- Marshmallow (*Althea off.*) (altheacoumarin)
- Meadowsweet (*Filipendula ulmaria*) (phenolic compounds)

Herbs to Help the Body Rebuild

- Hemp oil (*Cannabis Sativa*) (omega 3s and amino acids)

So, the bottom line is that there are a huge number of really good foods and herbs that are used for different aspects of arthritis – but again, find a good Herbalist who knows what she is doing and get the specific blend that your body needs. After all, we are all different. That uniqueness requires attention. You are much more likely to get that uniqueness attended to if you work with a Professional Health Practitioner. As opposed to working with a MD that only focuses on synthetic drugs and managing the symptoms of arthritis.

In addition, if you get a good Health Practitioner, that will do the research to see where the plants/herbs are grown, how they are harvested, and how they are prepared, you are going to be well looked after.

One note of caution: if they give you a 'tincture' made up just for you, it will usually taste awful. Be careful, if you complain they might give you a Chinese combination, and if you complain again, they will give you the worst, the East Indian ones. So, take your medicine and don't complain.

Chapter 12

Supplements for Arthritis

Okay, so we know pain killers are bad for you. We know that we need to eat healthy foods. But are there any supplements that can help?

There are a wide number. Let's look at some of them.

Good healthy fats

- Cod Liver oil
- Fish oil (will have different fish oils in it)
- Evening primrose oil
- Krill

Now you can buy a huge number of different Omega 3 supplements, but they do vary hugely.

- Whether they are synthetic or natural
- Where they are taken from if natural
- Plant or animal
- Where and how the plants were grown

- Whether the fish were farmed, whether in toxic water or in clean waters and what species
- The amount of fatty acid in each pill or capsule

Glutathione

I told you earlier about what a powerful compound Glutathione is in Chapter 8. And how important it is the immune system and to the anti-inflammatory processes in the body. So, we need to elaborate on glutathione here.

I also very simply explained what needs to happen in a cell in order to regulate and produce glutathione, which is what Dr Jane Gibson identifies in her book on glutathione. The following are the compounds that need to be incorporated into the diet and some examples of the foods that can provide these nutrients.

Glycine rich foods

- Garlic, chickpeas, beef, lamb, almond cashews, hemp

Methionine rich foods

- Kefir, broccoli, spinach, cod, halibut, salmon, garlic, almonds, cashews, hemp

Betaine rich foods

- Kefir, spinach, eggs, turmeric, beef, ham, chicken, beets

Methylation nutrients (foods rich in Vitamin B6, B9 & B12)

- Kefir, dark green leafy vegetables, quinoa, chicken, beef, lamb, beets

Cysteine rich foods

- Kefir, milk, yogurt, eggs, quinoa, bananas, garlic, onions, white/yellow beans, hemp, red peppers

Selenium rich foods

- Broccoli, spinach, seafood, oats, chickpeas, beef, cashews, hemp, chia

Sulfur rich foods

- Broccoli, collards, kale, seafood, rye, garlic, hemp, cabbage

Vitamin B6 rich foods

- Kefir, broccoli, spinach, salmon, tuna, avocado, cashews, hemp, beets

Vitamin B9/choline rich foods

- Yogurt, asparagus, broccoli, eggs, salmon, citrus fruits, beans, hemp, beets, Brussel sprouts

Vitamin B12 rich foods

- Cheese, eggs, sardines, shellfish, bran, beef

Serrapeptase

Serrapeptase is an enzyme that comes from silkworms. When the silkworm breaks through the cocoon, it needs something to break through the hard covering and the Serrapeptase is released to do that. If you are interested, it is a proteolytic enzyme which means that it breaks down protein.

Research has shown that Serrapeptase will break down unwanted/unneeded cellular structure in our bodies and helps with inflammation. A lot of people get a lot of relief with Serrapeptase.

If you want more information on Serrapeptase, you might want to look up Dr. Hans Nieper who identified it AND you might be interested in the research that shows it can also be used for the following:

- Causes varicose veins to shrink;
- Clear away arterial blockage;
- Decreases inflammation;
- Dissolves blood clots;
- Eliminates some types of tumors; and
- Removing arterial plaque.

But like most research there is controversy. We have to also realize that a lot of the controversy depends on who is funding the study and what they want to prove. If you want the funding to keep coming, you will end up proving what the funders want to hear.

Remember what I told you about the Editor-in-Chiefs of the big prestigious medical journals.

But this Grandma is not going into the statistical analysis and explain correlational versus causal or Manovas versus Canonicals, or or or. So, I go to those who are experts in the research and design and look for their current understandings of the nutrients required in the body.

And I go to the Professional Health Practitioners to get their advice.

Once nice simple article that has references and was written by a physician is "Health Benefits of Serrapeptase" by the Global Healing Center.[14]

Chapter 13

Creating Your Own Healthy Water

Now previously we discussed water and pH and how much you should drink. We also discussed how water can be full of toxins, especially if it has a low pH.

There are a number of beautiful water systems out there that you can purchase, like a Kangan Water System. But if you don't have the funds to buy a really good system, then here are some general guidelines for making your own.

1) Pour your tap water into a container and leave it overnight – most of the chlorides and fluorides will evaporate into the air.

2) Put the water into a blender and blend it for about a minute – this sort of impacts on water like a waterfall does. It will break up the clusters of H20 molecules we were talking about and of course, we only want small clusters of H20 molecules.

Now the theory here is that most of the toxins in the clusters are heavy and consequently will fall when the clusters are breaking up. So, we should leave the last ¼ of water in the blender

3) Purchase some alkalizing mineral drops from a health food store – we want water with alkalizing minerals in it – put in a couple of drops and voila – now you have a much cleaner water with a good pH and with alkalizing minerals. It costs virtually nothing AND we didn't pollute our environment with plastic bottles.

By the way, bottled water is often worse than tap water – make sure you check and don't just assume that it is healthy because it is bottled water.

Chapter 14

Tricks to Help You Manage the Pain Until You Resolve the Problem

The Gibsons gave me the following few home tricks that can often help manage arthritic pain. They are simple and easy. They are non-addictive. They have no horrible side-effects. So, they are always worth a try and they work for most people.

Trick #1

This one is from the bathroom: take a bar of Ivory soap. You may need two. Make sure there are no colorants or scents, just plain Ivory soap. Place them between the sheets in your bed. Just allow them to float around your body at night.

Apparently, they have recently discovered that it has something to do with the tallow that the soap is made from. Somehow it draws out the inflammation. I can tell you that when I used it, the bars of soap would sometimes be hot in the morning. But it sure worked. Good luck to you.

Trick #2

The second trick is from the kitchen. Take a bowl of golden raisins. Make sure it is not the black ones. Pour enough gin into the bowl to cover the raisins and cover with a cheesecloth. Wait for a couple of days until the raisins have soaked up the gin and then take 7-10 raisins a day.

Apparently, there is a chemical reaction between the terpenes, the Vitamin C, oleanic acids and phenols. Did you know that gin comes from juniper berries? Anyways the resulting chemical reaction makes a good pain killer.

Again, they are non-addictive. Well, they might be if you were an alcoholic, I guess. But otherwise, they are safe. No horrible side effects. And again, a lot cheaper than the prescription medications and more useful for most than the OTCs.

Chapter 15

Conclusions

Well, that is my story. I have shared with you:

- What can cause arthritis;
- What arthritis can cause;
- Scary facts about pain killers;
- How to solve the arthritis; and
- How to manage the pain while you are solving the arthritis

The one final thing I would strongly suggest is to find a good *health* practitioner and eliminate your arthritis and only use a symptom manager when you absolutely need to.

Choose to live a full and abundant life. All the very best to you, whatever you chose to do.

Grandma Mary

References

AGEs

www.todaysdietitian.com/newarchives/030314p10.
shtml

www.ncbi.nlm.nih.gov/pmc/articles/PMC4648888

Death by Medicine

www.webdc.com/pdfs/deathbymedicine.pdf

www.youtube.com/watch?v=RwCUDCQMLwY

archive.org/details/DeathByMedicine

EWG

www.EWG.org

EMFs

www.ncbi.nlm.nih.gov/pubmed/1397839

www.ncbi.nlm.nih.gov/pubmed/19398310

FDA Big Pharma & Lawsuits

https://www.lawyersandsettlements.com/articles/drugs-medical/fda_lawsuit-00192.html#.VmTWsnarS00

www.zerohedge.com/news/2015-02-18/nyu-professor-uncovers-how-fda-systematically-covers-fraud-misconduct-drug-trials

www.activistpost.com/2015/07/fda-does-big-pharmas-dirty-work-again.html

Relative risk versus absolute risk

proteinpower.com/drmike/2013/12/30/absolute-risk-versus-relative-risk-need-know-difference/

scienceblog.cancerresearchuk.org/2013/03/15/absolute-versus-relative-risk-making-sense-of-media-stories/

Teeth and Dr Weston Price

www.westonaprice.org/health-topics/weston-a-price-dds/

www.endalldisease.com/how-do-root-canals-cause-cancer/

arealfoodlover.wordpress.com/2012/04/15/how-i-remineralized-my-tooth-cavity-without-dentistry/

Vaccinations and Immunizations

vaccines.procon.org/

Water and Dr Pollock

www.structuredwaterunit.com/articles/structuredw
ater/dr-gerald-pollack-and-structured-water-science

Members of the Entwined Book Project

Smiths: Married for 23 years at the age of 24 and 25, October 25

Name: Maria, 47
Book: A Love that Crosses Time
Issue: Adrenal Fatigue
Character: Realtor that is a go getter, but family is most important; loves husband dearly

Name: Duncan, 48
Book: A Book for Men: How to Create a Good Marriage
Issue: Enlarged left ventricle
Character: Devoted husband and father

Name: Jessie, 20, daughter
Book: Female Sexuality
Issue: Diabetes
Character: University student, initially wants to be an MD but moves into Real Medicine, boyfriend Steve

Name: Jasmine, 15, daughter
Book: A Time Travel Romance
Issue: Asthma
Character: Dancer, somewhat shy, boyfriend Nick

Name: John, 9, son
Book: How Aliens Would Interpret our Planet
Issue: Allergies
Character: Artist, loves Granddad

Friends
Name: Steve, 20, Jessie's boyfriend
Book: How to Deal with Alcoholic Husbands
Issue: Alcoholic father
Character: University student, father alcoholic, submissive mother, avoids home-life, loves the Smith family

Name: Nick, 15, Jasmine's boyfriend
Book: Music, Sound & Other Energies for Healing
Character: Dancer, somewhat shy, Steve is like an older brother

Maria's Parents
Name: Grandma Mary
Book: Manage or Eliminate Arthritis
Issue: Arthritis
Character: Sweet; grandma type; adores grandpa

Name: Papa Johnny
Book: The Politics of Health
Issue: Dementia
Character: Funny old guy; set in his ways, but changing his mind

Maria's sister Carol and family
Name: Carol, Maria's sister
Book: Emotional Eating
Issue: Weight
Character: Kind of belligerent; but wants the best for her family
Husband George

Name: George, Maria's brother-in-law
Book: Covering Up Suicidal Thinking
Issue: Depression
Character: He's tries to be the man; but really isn't; not confident like Duncan; but holds his own with his wife Carol

Name: Tim, 19, Maria's nephew
Book: What it Feels Like NOT to be Understood
Issue: Paranoia
Character: Weak; not well developed; insecure, girlfriend Shelley

Name: Sherry, 15, Maria's niece
Book: A Romance About Gaining Self Control
Issue: Obsessive-Compulsive
Character: Struggles with control issues, boyfriend Randy

Name: Shelley
Book: Teen Age Empowerment
Issue:
Character: Tim's girlfriend

Maria's brother Dave and family
Name: Dave, Maria's brother
Book: When Enough is Enough
Issue: Divorce
Character: Dave compassionate man; gives too much; finally divorced bipolar abusive Joan

Grandma Mary's brother and family
Name: Dan
Book: How to Design Your Dream Home
Issue: High cholesterol, hyper -tension
Character: He's a good guy; but private; hasn't dated anyone since his wife Judy died years ago

Gibson family – own the Gibsons Clinic
Name: Dr Jim
Book: Personality Styles & Marriage
Character: Psychotherapist Social/outgoing; fun but wise, Julie's husband

Name: Julie
Book: A Book comparing East & West Religious Philosophies
Character: Physiotherapist, gentle; sweetheart; nurturing, Jim's wife

Name: Dr Jane
Book: A New Integrative Model for Cellular Healing
Character: Dr of Natural Medicine Academic; knows her stuff; confident in her knowledge Gibson's daughter

Name: Dr Daniel
Book: A Very Unique Cookbook
Character: PhD Nutrition, academic but has fun with food,
Gibson's son

Name: Nanny Sarah
Book: Romance and Cerebral Palsy
Character: Acupuncturist, gentle, nurturing, mothering, accommodating, Jim's mother

Name: Pappy
Book: Eliminating Autism
Character: Master Herbalist, fun, happy go lucky,
loves life, Jim's father

Endnotes

[1] http://www.collective-evolution.com/2015/05/16/editor-in-chief-of-worlds-best-known-medical-journal-half-of-all-the-literature-is-false/

[2] http://www.nybooks.com/articles/2009/01/15/drug-companies-doctorsa-story-of-corruption/

[3] https://proteinpower.com/drmike/2013/12/30/absolute-risk-versus-relative-risk-need-know-difference/

[4] (http://www.ewg.org/research/ewg-s-dirty-dozen-guide-food-additives/generally-recognized-as-safe-but-is-it)

[5] http://www.ncbi.nlm.nih.gov/pubmed/19398310

[6] https://www.lupusuk.org.uk/medical/gp-guide/diagnosis-of-lupus/associated-illnesses/drug-induced-lupus/

[7] https://www.webmd.com/lupus/what-is-drug-induced-lupus

[8] http://healthimpactnews.com/2012/medical-care-is-the-number-1-cause-of-death-in-the-u-s/

[9] www.Wikipedia.org/wiki/Microbiota

[10] http://educate-yourself.org/cn/rootcanalcoverup02apr04.shtml

[11] https://www.practicalpainmanagement.com/treatments/pharmacological/opioids/ask-expert-do-nsaids-cause-more-deaths-opioids

[12] https://www.ncbi.nlm.nih.gov/pmc/articles/PMC3748247/

[13] https://www.vox.com/science-and-health/2018/8/16/17698204/opioid-epidemic-overdose-deaths-2017

[14] http://www.globalhealingcenter.com/natural-health/health-benefits-of-serrapeptase/

www.ingramcontent.com/pod-product-compliance
Lightning Source LLC
Chambersburg PA
CBHW052209270326
41931CB00011B/2282